KE

Everyday Ketogenic Recipes To Lose Weight

By David D. Kings

Copyrights 2017 David D. Kings

No part of this book can be transmitted or reproduced in any form including print, electronic, photocopying, scanning, mechanical or recording without prior written permission from the author.

All information, ideas, and guidelines presented here are for educational purposes only. This book cannot be used to replace information provided with the device. All readers are encouraged to seek professional advice when needed.

This book is not intended to be a substitute for the medical advice of a licensed physician. The reader should consult with their doctor in any matters relating to his/her health.

David D. Kings

TABLE OF CONTENTS

TABLE OF CONTENTS..3

PREFACE...5

CHAPTER 1- KETO RECIPES FOR BREAKFAST...............9
- Mocha Chia Pudding...10
- Grain-free Hemp Heart Porridge..............................13
- Egg Porridge...15
- Almond Joy Pancakes..18
- Keto French Toast Muffins.......................................21
- Baked Spiced Granola...24
- Keto Zucchini Breakfast Hash..................................27
- Roasted Tomato Shakshuka....................................30
- Zero Carbs Eggs Benedict.......................................32
- Avocado and Salmon Breakfast Boats....................37

CHAPTER 2- KETO RECIPES FOR LUNCH......................41
- Chicken Salad – Low Carb Southern Goodness...........41
- Egg Salad Sandwiches..44
- Keto Caesar Salad...48
- Crispy Flourless Crab Cakes...................................52
- Low Carb Pizza..55
- Chicken Brocoli Casserole with cream cheese............58
- Easy Foil Chicken..60

CHAPTER 3- KETO RECIPES FOR DINNER......................65
- Caprese hasselback chicken...................................65
- Cabbage lasagna...69
- Low-Carb Zucchini Nachos......................................71
- Steak kebabs chimichurri sauce..............................74
- Keto Reuben Stromboli..76

Spinach Tomato Meatza Pizza - Paleo Low Carb..........79
Bacon cheeseburger casserole................................81
ABOUT THE AUTHOR..85
ONE LAST THING...87

PREFACE

There are many ways to diet using various kinds of philosophies. One proven method is to do low carbohydrate dieting. One form of low carb dieting is called ketogenic diets. This diet makes the body go into a state called ketosis. This state helps the body make sure it burns fat cells as carbohydrates are restricted so the body has to then turn to fat for its main source of energy. To ensure we can get to a ketogenic state, foods high in digestible carbohydrates should be replaced with foods low in carbohydrates.

As we limit the amount of carbohydrates and thus the calories from them we need to ensure we get enough calories from other sources, mainly protein and fat. One well known diet, Atkins, relies on this methodology during its "induction phase". This induction phase makes the participant eat a very low amount of carbohydrates whilst eating a high amount of protein and a moderate level of fat.

An excellent low carb ketogenic diet is called the cyclical ketogenic diet. The diet breaks down the amount of protein, carbs and fat into what is called macros. These macros help you distribute how much of each source of calories so you eat the right amount for each meal. The best breakdown for calories from protein, carbs and fat is a 65% fat, 30% protein, 5% carbohydrates ratio. The reason the diet is called a cyclical ketogenic diet is because we spend 5 days of the week doing a low carb phase and then the next two days is a high carb, or carb up, phase.

To work out how much to eat per day we start with by working out your maintenance calories which is roughly your weight, in lbs, multiplied by 13. Subtract 500 from this number to get your target calories per day. Using an example, a woman who weighs 145lbs works out her calories per day to be 1385 calories.

To work out the amount of protein calories per day to consume we need to multiply your weight by 30%. Using the example again, the amount of calories for protein would be 415.5 calories. We divide this by 4, as protein has 4 calories per gram, to work out how many grams per day to consume. The daily amount of protein for our example is 104 grams of protein. We do a similar calculation for the amount of fat required. You multiply your weight by 65% and then divide the number by the amount of calories per gram of fat, in this case it is 9, as there are 9 calories per gram. For our example the amount of fat in grams per day to eat is 100 grams. Finally the amount of carbs is worked out in a similar fashion. Multiply your weight by 5% then divide by 4. Using our example again the result is 17 grams of carbohydrates per day.

We now have the macros that tell us how many grams of each type of food we require per day on the low carb phase. A woman who weighs 145lbs requires 104 grams of protein, 100 grams of fat and 17 grams of carbohydrates. During the carb up phase try to have less than 50 grams of fat each day, about 150 grams of carbs and the same amount of protein you have during the week. Using this knowledge and information, you can then start preparing your low carb recipes following the different recipes information provided in this book and start planning a daily or weekly meal time table.

After starting the diet using these macros, about 3 days in, ketosis should start taking effect. This can be confirmed by using a product called Ketostix which measures the levels of ketones in your urine. Symptoms can be feeling groggy and less energy but after few days your energy levels pick up and you should feel great. Try and take a multi-vitamin supplement every day. Try and get in exercise a few times a week but do not overexert yourself by keeping cardio to a minimum. Please note do not undertake any new diets without properly discussing them with your medical practitioner.

CHAPTER 1- KETO RECIPES FOR BREAKFAST

Best Keto Breakfast Recipes For You!

Tell me the truth...is breakfast not your favorite meal of the day?

Well, it is for me. I wake up looking forward to some delicious food to start my day!

But a great breakfast should also have couple of very important features:

It should stabilize your blood sugars for the day, so you don't crash after an hour

It should provide you with plenty of good nutrients!

So here are some of my very favorite recipes to start the day! They are not all strictly Keto, some are low carb, but you can use them within a keto diet by distributing your carbs wisely.

Mocha Chia Pudding

This is a Herbal Coffee and Cacao Nibs Mocha Chia Pudding!

Why? Because if you are experiencing adrenal fatigue like so many people are nowadays, caffeine might not be the best thing for you.

Me? Not only I used to have adrenal fatigue and had to be off caffeine in general, but I am also hyper-sensitive to it!

"Caffeine is metabolized by the liver using the enzyme. The ability to produce this enzyme is regulated by the CYP1A2 gene. Slight changes in the DNA sequence of this gene determine how efficiently a person can metabolize caffeine and thus eliminate it from the body.

Some people genetically produce very little of this enzyme while others produce a large amount. The majority of humans are somewhere in the middle."

Using herbal coffee instead

Herbal coffee can be pretty much as tasty as the real deal!

I really like this Ayurvedic Roast!

Ayurvedic Roast is a 100% Certified Organic herbal coffee substitute that tastes like real coffee with no caffeine. Brews like coffee, drinks like coffee, without the edge and side effects of caffeine. It is the best tasting herbal coffee alternative currently available, and includes three antioxidant, adaptogenic, and immunity-enhancing organic ayurvedic herbs.

A Breakfast or a Treat.

When I created this pudding I wanted something like a treat, but cold, and flavorful and nutritious. I am a bit tired of eating fat bombs all the time, so I wanted to try something different.

By the way the cacao nibs also contain a bit of caffeine, just enough for a kick but not enough to keep me up all night!

Chia seeds are great as they have a fabulous nutritional profile: 100 grams of dried chia seeds contain 490 calories, of which 38 whopping grams of fiber, 16 grams of protein and 31 grams of fat. And ONLY 6 grams of net carbs. That makes it 76% fat, 17.4% protein and 6.6% carbs (mostly fiber!)

It's the perfect keto food!

To that wonderful nutrition you basically only need to add some matchingly good flavors and we are in business!

Mocha Chia Pudding

Serves: 2 servings

Serving size: 1 serving

Calories: 257

Fat: 20.25

Net Carbs: 2.25 NET

Fiber: 11.5

Protein: 7gr

Recipe type: DESSERT

Prep time: 5 mins

Cook time: 30 minutes

Total time: 35 mins

Ingredients

2 tbs herbal coffee

⅓ cup (55 gr) dry chia seeds

⅓ cup coconut cream - undiluted

1 tbsorganic vanilla extract

1 tbs Swerve

2 tbs (15 gr) Cacao nibs

Instructions

Brew a strong herbal coffee simmering 2 tbs of herbal blend with 2 cups of water for 15 minutes or until liquid is reduced to about 1 cup.

Strain the herbal coffee and blend in coconut cream, vanilla extract and swerve.

Add chia seeds and cacao nibs and stir well all together.

Place in serving containers and chill for minimum 30 minutes before serving.

You can add some additional herbal coffee to the pudding when serving and sprinkle with few cacao nibs to decorate.

Grain-free Hemp Heart Porridge

Recipe type: Vegan, Paleo, Gluten-free, Dairy-free, Sugar-free, Yeast-free, Corn-free, Grain-free, Egg-free, Low-Carb, Keto

Prep time: 2 minutes Cook time: 3 mins Total time: 5 mins

Serves: 1

A grain-free, keto porridge made with only nuts and seeds. Over 24 grams of fiber in every bowl, a hearty meal that's gluten-free, dairy-free, vegan, low-carb and paleo.

Ingredients
1 cup non-dairy milk
½ cup Manitoba Harvest Hemp Hearts
2 tablespoons freshly ground flax seed
1 tablespoon chia seeds
1 tablespoon xyltiol or 5 drops alcohol-free stevia
¾ teaspoon pure vanilla extract
½ teaspoon ground cinnamon
¼ cup crushed almonds or almond flour
Toppings
3 Brazil nuts
1 tablespoon Manitoba Harvest Hemp Hearts

Instructions

Add all ingredients but the ground almonds and toppings to a small saucepan. Stir until combined, then heat over medium heat, just until it begins to boil lightly. No need to cover.

Once bubbling lightly, stir once over and leave to cook for another 1-2 minutes.

Remove from the heat, stir in crushed almonds, and drop into a bowl. Top with toppings and eat immediately.

Notes

Making Ahead: I have not tried making this keto recipe ahead of time and eating it later. I'm not sure if it would get too sticky?

Nut-free: If you can't do nuts, simply replace the ground almonds with crushed sunflower seeds or pumpkin seeds.

Digestion: If you're sensitive to nuts and seeds, you could try soaking the ingredients beforehand.

Egg Porridge

Here is an interesting (and satiating!) option for those who are after porridge for breakfast but are lacking proper gluten-free and ketogenic porridge recipes. This sweet, creamy and rich breakfast "porridge" keeps you satisfied for hours.

This creation is quite close to scrambled eggs but grainier, creamier and sweeter. In fact, when spiced with cinnamon, it resembles rice porridge that we eat during Christmas time. It also reminds me of Milchreis ("milk rice"), that Germans eats any time.

If your daily quota of carbs allows, top this porridge with berries or slices of apples or peaches. Berries are highly recommended because of their valuable nutrients.

TIPS FOR MAKING THE EGG PORRIDGE

This whole recipe is based on the curdling of eggs. The curdles are tiny and create a porridge-like effect. There are not that many occasions where curdling is preferred, but here curdling is a must!

This porridge is very easy and quick to make — perfect for busy mornings — and it's almost foolproof. (How could you go wrong with curdling, when it anyway happens so easily, also when you last wish it?) The most important thing is to mix the egg and cream mixture all the time when heating, also along the bottom. Use low enough heat to ensure that the mixture doesn't burn to the bottom of the saucepan and doesn't get any brown color.

Ingredients

2 organic free-range eggs

1/3 cup = 80 ml organic heavy cream without food additives

2 packages NuStevia™ NoCarbs Blend™ OR your preferred sweetener to taste

2 tablespoons = 1 oz = 30 g grass-fed butter

to taste ground organic Ceylon cinnamon

Directions

Combine eggs, cream and the sweetener in a small bowl. Give the mixture a little whisk.

Melt the butter in a medium saucepan over medium-high heat. Don't let the butter get any brown color, but just melt. Turn the heat to the minimum once the butter is melted.

Add the egg and cream mixture. Cook, all the time mixing along the bottom until the mixture thickens and starts curdling.

When you see the first signs of curdling, i.e. those tiny grains, take the saucepan immediately from the heat. Now the porridge is ready!

Transfer the porridge in a serving bowl. Sprinkle plenty of cinnamon on top and serve immediately.

Almond Joy Pancakes

Almond Joy Pancakes (Gluten Free)
Prep Time
10 minutes
Cook Time
10 minutes
Total Time
20 minutes

Almond Joy Pancakes are made with coconut flour for a tasty gluten free breakfast treat.

Servings: 12

Calories: 266 kcal

Ingredients

1/2 cup coconut flour I use Bob's Red Mill

1/3 cup unsweetened shredded coconut

1/4 cup sweetener of choice I use Swerve Sweetener

1/2 tsp baking powder

1/2 tsp salt

6 large eggs

1/4 cup coconut oil melted

1/2 cup to 1 cup unsweetened almond milk

1 tsp almond extract

1/4 cup toasted slivered almonds

2 ounces 85 - 90% cacao chocolate finely chopped

Additional oil for the pan

US Measurements - Convert to Metric

Instructions

In a large bowl, whisk together coconut flour, shredded coconut, sweetener, baking powder and salt.

Stir in eggs, coconut oil, 1/2 cup of the almond milk, and the almond extract. Add additional almond milk as needed. Your batter should be thicker than traditional pancake batter, but not so thick that you can't pour it and spread it around the pan. Coconut flour batters also tend to thicken up as they sit so you can add additional milk partway through.

Stir in toasted almonds and chopped chocolate.

Heat a large skillet over medium heat and brush with additional coconut oil or another cooking oil. Scoop about 2 heaping tablespoons of batter onto skillet and spread into a 4-inch circle. Repeat until you can't fit any more pancakes into skillet (you should get 3 or 4 in).

Cook until the bottom is golden brown and the top is set around the edges. You will see little bubbles start to come up in the center of the pancake, a good sign that it's cooked enough to flip.

Flip and continue cooking until second side is golden brown. Remove from pan and keep warm. Repeat with remaining batter.

Nutrition Facts
Almond Joy Pancakes (Gluten Free)

Amount Per Serving (1 pancake)

Calories 266 Calories from Fat 153

% Daily Value*

Total Fat 17g 26%

Cholesterol 212mg 71%

Sodium 372mg 16%

Total Carbohydrates 17g 6%

Dietary Fiber 9g 36%

Protein 11g 22%

* Percent Daily Values are based on a 2000 calorie diet.

Keto French Toast Muffins

Come on, just admit it. You haven't had french toast in a while and you want it now. This is the perfect excuse to get that cinnamon-y, semi-crunchy, delicious taste.

You can put some twists of your own on this one for sure. Add maple extract or Walden Farms Maple Syrup. You can add allspice, clove, or any other spice you see fit and think would work well. My intentions was to keep this simple, so almost everyone could make this.

Keep in mind that I normally don't eat berries, but you can eat berries if you want, especially if it's only a few of them. The whipped cream is not as optional, though, and I highly recommend adding it to the muffins.

Yields 11 Total French Toast Muffins

The Preparation

- 6 large eggs
- 2/3 cup almond flour
- ¼ cup peanut butter
- ¼ cup heavy whipping cream
- ¼ cup crushed toasted almonds
- 2 tablespoons coconut oil
- 1 tablespoon unsalted butter
- 2 tablespoons erythritol
- 1 teaspoon cinnamon
- 1 teaspoon vanilla
- ½ teaspoon of salt
- ¼ teaspoon nutmeg
- 10 drops liquid Stevia

Per muffin, you'll be looking at 171 Calories, 16.3g Fats, 2g Net Carbs, and 6.9g Protein.

The Execution

Preheat oven to 350F.

Grind 1/4 Cup Almonds in the food processor and stick them in a pan on medium-high heat to toast. Make sure you keep an eye on them and stir as needed.

Mix together your almond flour, erythritol, cinnamon, salt, and nutmeg.

In a microwave safe bowl, add your coconut oil, butter and peanut butter, then microwave for 30-40 seconds to melt it.

Add your peanut butter, coconut oil, butter, eggs, vanilla, stevia, and heavy cream to the almond flour and mix well.

Fill cupcake tray with the batter, then top with toasted almonds.

Bake for 20-25 minutes, let cool for 5 minutes, then remove from cupcake tray and let cool for an additional 10-15 minutes. Serve with whipped cream.

Baked Spiced Granola

Ever since I gave up grains I missed my breakfast granola. I was determined to make a healthier low-carb and paleo-friendly alternative and created some of the best granola recipes.

This recipe uses less sweeteners but you can add more Eryhritol or stevia if you prefer a sweeter taste. Granola goes great with full-fat yogurt, cream, almond milk or coconut milk and it's great when topped with fresh or frozen berries. Looking for a snack? Put some granola in an airtight container and keep in your bag to have any time you feel hungry!

Nutritional values (per serving / ~ ½ cup)

Total Carbs 14.6 grams
Fiber 9 grams
Net Carbs 5.6 grams
Protein 16 grams
Fat 37.2 grams
of which Saturated 14.1 grams
Energy (calories) 434 kcal
Magnesium 126 mg (32%)
Potassium 441 mg (22%)

Macronutrient ratio: Calories from carbs (5.3%), protein (15.2%), fat (79.5%)

Ingredients (makes 8 servings)

Dry ingredients:
1 cup almonds, whole (140 g/ 4.9 oz)
½ cup macadamia nuts (65 g/ 2.3 oz)
½ cup pecan nuts (50 g/ 1.8 oz)
1 cup shredded dried coconut, unsweetened (75 g/ 2.6 oz)
1 cup flaked dried coconut, unsweetened (60 g/ 2.1 oz)
½ cup pumpkin seeds (60 g/ 2.1 oz)
¼ cup chia seeds, whole or ground (32 g/ 1.1 oz)
½ cup vanilla or plain whey protein or egg white protein powder (Jay Robb) or plant-based such as NuZest or ¼ cup powdered egg whites (50 g / 1.8 oz)
¼ cup Erythritol or Swerve or other healthy low-carb sweetener from this list (40 g/ 1.4 oz)
1 tbsp + 1 tsp pumpkin pie spice mix (you can make your own)
¼ tsp salt (I like pink Himalayan)

Wet ingredients:
½ cup pumpkin puree (you can make your own) (100 g / 3.5 oz)

1 large egg white, free-range or organic

¼ cup extra virgin coconut oil, melted (55 g / 1.9 oz)

10-15 drops liquid Stevia extract

One serving is about ½ cup of granola. The main reason I use two sweeteners in most of my recipes is that a combination of more sweeteners mask the aftertaste / bitterness of some of them. Ideally, use soaked & dehydrated nuts. Have a look at my post here to learn how and why you should do it

Instruction

Preheat the oven to 150 C / 300 F. Roughly chop the almonds, macadamia nuts and pecans and place them in a mixing bowl.

Add the shredded and flaked coconut, chia seeds, pumpkin seeds, protein powder (or powdered egg whites) and Erythritol.

Add the pumpkin spice mix and salt. Pour in the egg white, melted coconut oil and add stevia. Mix until well combined.

Add the pumpkin puree and mix well. If using canned pumpkin puree, make sure you opt for BPA-free product like this one.

Place the granola mixture on a baking tray and spread evenly over the surface. Keto Pumpkin Spiced Granola

Place in the oven and bake for 30-40 minutes or until crispy.

Once done, remove from the oven and set aside on a cooling rack. Once chilled, transfer into a jar or airtight container and keep at room temperature for up to a month. Serve with cream, yogurt, almond milk or coconut milk and enjoy!

Keto Zucchini Breakfast Hash

I love making any kind of hash and not just for breakfast. It's my go-to meal when I don't have time to cook or don't feel like cooking. It's quick and you won't need any special skills. Although I used zucchini, you can try any of your favourite veggies: brussels sprouts, turnips, kale, broccoli or cauliflower - all work great! Then, add some protein like bacon, minced meat or chicken and season with spices and herbs of your liking. Top with a fried egg or avocado and your hash is done!

Nutritional values (per serving)

Total Carbs 9.1 grams
Fiber 2.5 grams
Net Carbs 6.6 grams
Protein 17.4 grams
Fat 35.5 grams
of which Saturated 15.7 grams
Energy 423 kcal
Magnesium 53 mg (13% RDA)
Potassium 775 mg (39% EMR)
Macronutrient ratio: Calories from carbs (6%), protein (17%), fat (77%)

Ingredients (makes 1 serving)

- 1 medium zucchini (200 g/ 7.1 oz)
- 2 slices bacon (60 g/ 2.1 oz)
- ½ small white onion (30 g/ 1.1 oz) or 1 clove garlic
- 1 tbsp ghee or coconut oil
- 1 tbsp freshly chopped parsley or chives
- ¼ tsp salt (I like pink Himalayan)
- 1 large egg, free-range or organic on top (for AIP-friendly, egg-free alternative, top with ½ avocado instead)

Peel and finely chop the onion (or garlic) and slice the bacon.

Sweat the onion over a medium heat and add the bacon. Stir frequently and cook until lightly browned.

Meanwhile, dice the zucchini into medium pieces.

Add the zucchini to the pan and cook for 10-15 minutes. When done, remove from the heat and add chopped parsley.

Top with a fried egg or avocado. Enjoy!

Roasted Tomato Shakshuka

This dish comes to us from Tunisia and can be seen enjoyed all throughout the Middle East. It's essentially eggs poached in a sauce made of tomatoes and chili peppers. At first, you may be intimidated by how exotic it sounds, but the whole thing can be made in under 30 minutes! If you're bored of your usual scrambled eggs in the mornings, then this can be a great alternative.

You can choose to make your sauce from scratch if you have the time or have a really awesome recipe. We decided to cut down on some time and use one of our favorite marinara sauces.

For this recipe, we used chili peppers to add some authentic spice, but if you don't have any, feel free to get creative and add spice in different ways. Season with cayenne, red pepper flakes or just add your favorite hot sauce! And as always, add more pepper if you can take the heat!

MACROS PER SERVING:
- 490 Calories
- 34g of Fat
- 35g of Protein
- 4g of Net Carbs

Servings Prep Time Cook Time

1 serving 10 minutes 10 minutes

Servings: 1

Ingredients

1 cup marinara sauce

1 chili pepper

4 eggs

1 oz feta cheese

1/8 tsp cumin

salt

pepper

fresh basil

Instructions

Preheat the oven to 400°F.

Heat a small skillet on a medium flame with a cup of marinara sauce and some chopped chili pepper. Let the chili pepper cook for about 5 minutes in the sauce.

Crack and gently lower your eggs into the marinara sauce.

Sprinkle feta cheese all over the eggs and season with salt, pepper and cumin.

Using an oven mitt, place the skillet into your oven and bake for about 10 minutes. Now the skillet should be hot enough to continue cooking the food in the oven instead of heating itself up first.

Once the eggs are cooked, but still runny, take the skillet out with an oven mitt. Chop some fresh basil and sprinkle over the shakshuka. Enjoy straight out of the skillet but be careful- it will remain hot for some time! Enjoy!

Zero Carbs Eggs Benedict

Low carb style! Eggs are one of the most versatile foods on Earth! Fried, poached, boiled, emulsified, beaten, whipped, baked, separated, souffle or eaten raw- eggs are a must! They're full of fat and protein, with very little carbs, which makes them perfect for anyone on a ketogenic diet. The average large egg contains 5g of fat, 7g of protein and about 0.4g of carbs. Most nutrition labels round down on the carb count as it's minimal, but it's good to note. They are also good sources of choline and lutein, both important nutrients for brain and eye health.

When buying eggs, it's important to know where they're coming from (as much as you can infer from the package). Egg cartons these days are full of labels and certifications claiming their chickens are well taken care of. Some of those claims are simple marketing tactics and mean nothing; it's important to recognize them.

if you don't have any oopsie rolls on hand, here's the recipe! You can make a big batch of them and used them for savory and even sweet dishes. They're a keto staple!

Once you've got a dozen eggs that came from a good source, you're ready to make some delicious and healthy low carb Eggs Benedict. If you're on an Egg Fast, this recipe is perfect! Perhaps the Canadian bacon doesn't follow the rules entirely, but that can easily be omitted.

MACROS PER SERVING:
- 497 Calories
- 38.1g of Fat
- 30.3g of Protein
- 2.4g of Carbs

Servings Prep Time Cook Time
2 servings 10 minutes 15 minutes
Servings:
2

Ingredients
Eggs Benedict
4 Oopsie rolls
4 eggs
4 slices Canadian bacon
1 tbsp white vinegar
1 tsp chives
Hollandaise Sauce
2 egg yolks

2 tbsp butter

1 tsp lemon juice

1 pich salt

1 pinch paprika

Instructions

Start off making a quick hollandaise sauce. Separate 2 eggs and whisk the yolks in a glass bowl until they've doubled in volume. Add a squish of lemon juice.

Set a pot of water to boil. You need only about an inch of water set to simmer.

Begin melting some butter to later add to the sauce to emulsify.

Using a double boiler (or the glass bowl set on top of the simmering water) start to whisk the lemony egg yolks rapidly. You will see they will become thicker the more you whisk and gently heat.

Pour in the melted butter slowly all while still whisking, Be careful not to heat so much the eggs begin to cook too quick and turn into scrambled eggs!

The hollandaise sauce should be thick enough to coat the back of a spoon when lifted out.

When the hollandaise sauce is done, take it away from the heat and leave aside. Season with salt and paprika. If it cools and thickens too much, simply add a teaspoon of water and whisk to make it spoonable again.

Onto the eggs! To poach your eggs, set a pot of water to boil. About 3 inches of water here.

Once the water comes to a boil, reduce it to simmer and add some salt and a tablespoon on white vinegar.

Create a whirlpool in the water with a wooden spoon by stirring around a few times in one direction.

Crack an egg into a teacup and gently lower into the whirlpool you've created. Don't drop the egg in, rather lower the cup into the water and let it out.

Let the egg cook for about 2-4 minutes. You want these eggs to be pretty runny.

Lift the egg gently with a spatula and let it rest on a paper towel lined plate. Do the same with the rest of the eggs.

Fry up the Canadian bacon if you'd like. We like it a little crispy and warm.

Top 4 oopsie rolls with the Canadian bacon and gently place a poached egg onto each slice of bacon.

Spoon about a tablespoon of hollandaise sauce onto each poached eggs and top with some salt and pepper and chopped chives. Enjoy right away!

Avocado and Salmon Breakfast Boats

More than ever I realize how important breakfast is in the daily scope of things, especially regarding your blood glucose levels. You can stray a bit for lunch, but really breakfast and dinner are your two pillars for building the foundation of a level and healthy blood glucose.

You will see a lot of cheese and bacon in most ketogenic, low carb breakfast recipes. As the purpose of this blog is to bring you HEALTHY food, I am trying a bit harder.

Saturated fat and weight loss

Eating a lot of saturated fat during the adaptation phase of the ketogenic diet will result in a slower rate weight loss, as your body is trying to get rid of it's own fat.

Also do not forget that the meat of feedlot raised animals contains high levels of Omega 6's, which raise inflammation in the body.

Wild caught salmon is a good healthy fat alternative, so are organic avocados. Of course, if you can find pastured beef and pork, that is a good option too, really worth investing the extra dollar.

Here is a simple but yummy recipe for you, with an even simpler variation.

> Nutrition Information
> Serves: 1
> Serving size: 1
> Calories: 525
> Fat: 48 gr
> Saturated fat: 10 gr
> Net Carbs: 4 gr
> Sodium: 439 mg
> Protein: 19 gr

Recipe type: BREAKFAST
Cuisine: AMERICAN
Prep time: 5 mins
Total time: 5 mins

Ingredients

1 ripe organic avocado (about 100 grams or 2.5 oz)
60 grams (2 oz) of wild caught smoked salmon
30 grams (1 oz) of fresh, soft goat cheese
2 tablespoons of organic extra virgin olive oil
the juice of 1 lemon
a pinch of celtic sea salt

Instructions

Cut the avocado in two and remove the seed

In a small food processor mix the rest of the ingredients until coarsely chopped.

Place the resulting cream inside the avocado.

Serve immediately.

VARIATION

Cut the avocado in small cubes.

Cut the salmon in small pieces.

Mix the two together.

Add the goat cheese and the rest of the ingredients and blend well.

CHAPTER 2- KETO RECIPES FOR LUNCH

Many of my readers and patients work outside the house, some even have to commute for hours, just to come to an area which is a complete nutritional wasteland.

What do you do when restaurant food offers no good options for your keto lunch? You make one of these easy keto lunches and bring it to work the next day!! It's a great way to eat better, save money, and stay on the plan!

Some of these recipes do contain dairy, so please keep in mind that they could be modified in case you are Keto-Paleo and sensitive to dairy!

Salads & Sandwiches Recipes

Chicken Salad – Low Carb Southern Goodness

Try this delicious and moreish, comfort, chicken salad. It's terrifically low carb and if you have the time, is even tastier with homemade Basic Mayonnaise and if you want a sandwich, whip up some of Fluffy Chix Cook's Basic Revolution-ary Focaccia Bread or Rolls, low carb keto and Atkins Induction Friendly.

Prep Time: 10 minutes

Total Time: 10 minutes

Yield: 1 1/2 cups (3 servings)

Serving Size: 1/2 cup

Calories per serving: 283

Fat per serving: 23g

Ingredients

1 celery ribs, minced finely
1 green onion, minced finely
2 tablespoons Italian parsley, minced finely
5 ounces roasted chicken breast meat, minced finely
1 large hard-boiled eggs, chopped finely

1/2 tablespoon Vlasic Homestyle Dill Relish

1/8 teaspoon granulated garlic

1/3 cup mayonnaise (Hellmann's or Duke's})—or Basic Mayonnaise

1 teaspoon Country Dijon Mustard

kosher salt

fresh ground black pepper

Instructions

Make this gorgeous chicken salad by hand or use the food processor to make work even easier. Place celery, onions, and parsley in the bowl of a food processor. Pulse until veggies are extremely fine. Transfer to a mixing bowl. Add chunks of chicken white meat. Pulse until very fine. Transfer to mixing bowl. Grate peeled hard-boiled egg on the largest grater on a box grater or split and pulse in food processor until very fine but still separate piece. Transfer to mixing bowl.

Add remaining ingredients through Country Dijon Mustard. Mix well using a large spoon or spatula. Season to taste with kosher or coarse grain sea salt and freshly ground black pepper. Mix again to thoroughly incorporate. Keep refrigerated in an airtight container up to 1 week.

Notes

Use any leftover, cooked, boneless, skinless, chicken on hand. Rotisserie, grilled breasts or thighs, boiled, roasted, microwaved-steamed, or even smoked and barbecued, etc, all work fabulously well in this recipe. The point of this chicken salad is that it's a convenient and tasty way to repurpose Lucky Leftover chicken. The original recipe calls for scraped white onion, but I've come to prefer the taste to green onions or scallions as we call them in Texas.

Serving Ideas Serve on low carb bread or buns, in low carb wraps, or in lettuce boats. It's great plonked on top of a salad. Delish!

Nutritional Information

Per ½ Cup: 283 Calories; 23g Fat (75.0% calories from fat); 16g Protein; 1g Carbohydrate; 0.33g Dietary Fiber; 176mg Cholesterol; 0.67g Effective Carbs

Egg Salad Sandwiches

This Keto Egg Salad makes the perfect lunch option or in smaller portions a delicious high-fat side. I am sharing this recipe with the nutrition info both with and without veggies. If you opt for a veggie-free version, you can enjoy this keto egg salad with NO carbs! I like to get my veggies in any way I can, but know not everyone loves them as much as I do.

Keto Egg Salad: Ingredients

Keto Egg Salad Recipe - I LOVE egg salad and this recipe is loaded with flavor! Egg salad with peppers, celery, mayo, mustard, and more. | ketosizeme.com

- 8 Large Eggs
- 2 Celery Stalks
- 2 Green Onion Stalks (tops only)
- 1 Green Pepper
- 1 tsp Yellow Mustard
- 2/3 Cup Mayonnaise
- Optional:
- Salt
- Paprika

Keto Egg Salad: Directions

Boil Eggs -Place eggs in the bottom of a pot and fill with cold water. Bring the water to a rolling boil and turn off the burner. Cover pot with a lid and let them cook for 15 minutes. Remove eggs and place in a bowl of ice water. Allow to cool completely and peel.

Chop celery, green onions, and green pepper.

Peel and cut boiled eggs

In a bowl add yolks, mayo, and mustard and mix well with a spoon.

Stir in your chopped whites, green pepper, celery, and green onion.

Top with paprika and salt (to taste). This is optional
Serves 1/2 Cup

Keto Egg Salad: Nutrition
This is for one serving (makes 4 1/2 cup servings)

Calories: 439
Total Fat: 41g
Cholesterol: 277mg

Sodium: 267mg

Potassium: 226mg

Carbohydrates: 4g – 1g Fiber = 3 NET CARBS

Dietary Fiber 1g

Sugars: 1g

Protein: 12g

Keto Egg Salad Without The Veggies:

I always have to make half of the recipe above for my husband. He hates peppers, onions, and celery so this is the version I make for him.

Ingredients:

4 Large Eggs (Boiled, Peeled, and Sliced)

1/3 Cup Mayo

1/2 tsp Mustard

Follow the instructions above.

Calories: 404

Fat: 41 grams

Carbs: 0

Protein: 12 grams

Keto Caesar Salad

This low carb caesar salad is one of my favourite weeknight meals. It is forgiving, tasty and filling and left overs make fantastic lunches the next day. It is also easily scaleable to feed a crowd if you are entertaining on a hot night.

I always keep a dozen boiled eggs in the fridge in their shells, which often leads to many Caesar salads!

You can make your own caesar dressing using the recipe below, or do some research into a store bought caesar dressing. I personally use Zoosh Caesar Dressing when I am running short on time or don't have the ingredients available.

Chicken Caesar Salad
A quick and satisfying salad, high in protein and flavor! On the table in 30 minutes.

Prep Time 10 minutes
Cook Time 15 minutes
Total Time 25 minutes
Servings 4
Calories 633 kcal

Ingredients

250 grams chicken breast

1 tablespoon dried oregano

1 clove garlic or ½ teaspoon of crushed garlic

25 grams parmesan cheese shaved

2 large eggs hard boiled and sliced

100 grams bacon

1/4 teaspoon salt and pepper

1 Cos lettuce

Caesar Dressing Ingredients - or use a store bought low carb dressing

2 egg yolks

2 teaspoons Dijon mustard

1 clove garlic chopped

4 anchovies optional, chopped

1 tablespoon red wine vinegar

3/4 cup olive oil

Optional

Avocado, red onion, cherry tomatoes

Instructions

To make the dressing

Place egg yolks, mustard, garlic, anchovies and vinegar in a blender or a jug if you have a bar mix/immersion blender and mix thoroughly to combine. With the motor running, slowly add the olive oil until dressing thickens. Season with salt and pepper. Cover and refrigerate until ready to serve. This is great to prepare ahead, and then just throw it all together at dinner time!

To make the salad

Place the eggs in a small saucepan of cold water. Put over high heat until a boil commences, then turn down the heat to medium and cook for 4 minutes. Run under cold water until cool enough to handle, and then peel the shells and dry, placing to one side.

Dice the bacon and fry in a non-stick frying pan until crispy. Remove from the pan and drain on paper towel, leaving the bacon grease in the pan.

Dice the chicken. Using the bacon frying pan, very lightly fry the garlic until fragrant. Toss in the chicken and oregano and cook through.

Season lightly with salt and pepper. Place to one side.

To serve, loosely cut the lettuce leaves (or leave them whole if you like!) and scatter around the bacon and chicken. Grate the parmesan cheese (I like to use my vegetale peeler to get nice strip and scatter over the salad.

Cut the egg in quarters and drizzle with the Caesar dressing.

Nutrition Facts
Amount Per Serving
Calories 633 Calories from Fat 522
% Daily Value*
Total Fat 58g 89%
Saturated Fat 12g 60%
Cholesterol 253mg 84%
Sodium 557mg 23%
Potassium 357mg 10%
Total Carbohydrates 1g 0%
Protein 24g 48%
Vitamin A 18.8%
Vitamin C 1.8%
Calcium 10.9%
Iron 8.3%

Easy bites:

Crispy Flourless Crab Cakes

The secret to making crisp crab cakes that don't fall apart without flour or bread is to drain the crab mixture very well. It can be made a day ahead and the cakes can be formed and refrigerated for several hours before cooking.

1 pound of jumbo lump crabmeat
2 green onions, white and light-green parts, finely chopped
1/4 cup flat-leaf parsley, chopped
1/4 cup fresh cilantro, finely chopped
1 tsp seeded and minced jalapeno pepper. optional
1 tsp Worcestershire sauce
1 tsp of fresh lemon juice
1 tsp Old Bay seasoning
1/2 tsp powdered mustard
1 large egg
1/2 cup real mayonnaise, home-made preferred
A pinch of salt
2 tbsp light olive oil (not extra-virgin), bacon fat, or other high heat fat.

Go through crab meat and pick out any bits of shell or cartilage, leaving lumps intact as much as possible. Place picked crab in a large bowl.

Add green onions, parsley, cilantro, jalapeno, Worcestershire sauce, lemon juice, Old Bay, and mustard to bowl. Carefully fold in without breaking up the lumps of crab meat.

Beat egg in a second bowl; add mayonnaise and mix well. Gently fold into crab mixture and place in a strainer. Set strainer over a large bowl. Cover strainer and bowl with plastic wrap and refrigerate for several hours or overnight.

Discard liquid and shape mixture into 6 cakes. They should be about 3 inches in diameter and about 1/2-inch thick. Cover and refrigerate until ready to cook.

Place a baking sheet in oven and preheat to 200°F.

Heat half the oil in a large skillet over medium heat until it shimmers in the pan. Place half the crab cakes in the skillet and cook without moving for 3 minutes or until the bottoms are well browned. Turn them over with a wide spatula. Cook for another 3 minutes until the second side is brown. Transfer to heated baking sheet and put in oven to keep warm until the remaining cakes are cooked.

Wipe out skillet and add the rest of the oil. Heat oil as before and repeat the cooking process. Serve warm.

TIPS:

Many stores sell fresh crab in 1-pound cans that can be stored in the refrigerator for quite a long time. I'm not sure I want to know how they do that, but it is very good, with large, meaty chunks of crab, and it is also relatively inexpensive compared to the fresh crab at the fish counter.

Be sure to get "real" mayonnaise. It will have real eggs and no sugar. Better yet, make your own fresh mayonnaise. The nutrition data shown is for purchased real mayonnaise, such as Hellman's, Best Food's, or Duke's.

Some of the fat used for frying will be left in the pan. The amount left in the crab cakes is estimated in the nutrition data.

Yield: 6 servings.

Per each crab cake: 257 calories; 19.4g protein; 18.5 g fat; 0.3g fiber; 0.6g net carbs

NOTE:

"Light" olive oil has the same number of calories as other olive oil but it is more refined, giving it a higher smoke point than extra-virgin and making it a better choice for frying and high-temperature cooking. Extra virgin olive oil is best reserved for salad dressings and quick sautéing. Other oils that can take the heat without being damaged include natural lard, beef and poultry fat, bacon fat, and some nut oils.

Low Carb Pizza

69% Fat
27% Protein
4% Carbs
8 g carbs / serving

Ingredients

Crust

4 eggs

175 g shredded cheese, preferably mozzarella or provolone

3 tablespoons tomato paste

1 teaspoon dried oregano

120 g shredded cheese

50 g pepperoni

olives

For serving

150 g leafy greens

olive oil

sea salt

Instructions

Preheat the oven to 400°F (200°C).

Beat the eggs and blend in 6 ounces (170 g) of cheese. Spread the cheese and egg batter on a baking sheet lined with parchment paper. You can form two round circles or just make one large rectangular pizza. Bake in the oven for 15 minutes until the pizza crust turns golden. Remove and let cool for a minute or two.

Increase the oven temperature to 450°F (225°C).

Spread tomato paste on the crust and sprinkle oregano on top. Top with 4 ounces cheese and place the pepperoni and olives on top.

Bake for another 5-10 minutes or until the pizza has turned a golden brown color.

Serve with a salad.

Tip!

Go ahead and try sun-dried tomato pesto or a jar of spaghetti sauce or pizza sauce, but make sure there is no added sugar.

Low-carb topping options are endless: bacon, salami, mushrooms, blue cheese, shredded chicken, sautéed onions, feta cheese... you know what you like!

Warm up:

Chicken Brocoli Casserole with cream cheese

A very quick to prepare low carb chicken casserole that is made completely from scratch without relying on a canned soup base.

Prep Time 10 minutes
Cook Time 35 minutes
Total Time 45 minutes
Servings 8 people
Calories 270 kcal

Ingredients
1 1/2 pounds boneless chicken breast
2 tablespoons olive oil
2 tablespoons butter
3 cloves garlic
1 tablespoon dried minced onion

salt and pepper to taste

1/2 teaspoon tarragon

6.5 ounces can mushroom sliced

1/2 cup white cooking wine or a few tablespoons of lemon juice

8 ounces cream cheese

1/3 cup sour cream

1 cup chicken broth

1 lb broccoli florets

1/2 cup parmesan cheese 1 3/4 ounces

Get Ingredients Powered by Chicory

Instructions

Slice chicken into bite sized pieces.

Cook chicken with garlic and onion in olive oil and butter until no longer pink.

Add remaining ingredients.

Cook and stir over medium heat for about 10 minutes. Pour into 9×13 casserole dish.

Sprinkle with Parmesan cheese.

Bake at 350 degrees F for 20-25 minutes.

Nutrition Facts

Chicken Broccoli Casserole

Amount Per Serving (197 g)

Calories 270 Calories from Fat 192

% Daily Value*

Total Fat 21.3g 33%

Saturated Fat 11.1g 56%

Cholesterol 62mg 21%

Sodium 297mg 12%

Potassium 397mg 11%

Total Carbohydrates 6.9g 2%

Dietary Fiber 1.8g 7%

Sugars 1.8g

Protein 12.2g 24%

Vitamin A 19%

Vitamin C 86%

Calcium 15%

Iron 9%

* Percent Daily Values are based on a 2000 calorie diet.

Easy Foil Chicken

Prep Time: 10 minutes

Cook Time: 1 hour, 30 minutes

Total Time: 1 hour, 40 minutes

Yield: 36 ounces white meat chicken

Serving Size: 3-4 ounces cooked meat

Calories per serving: 69 kcals/ounce

Fat per serving: 3g F

Ingredients

3 pounds bone-in chicken breasts or thighs—or whole chickens
1 tablespoon Better Than Bouillon Beef
1 tablespoon granulated garlic
2 tablespoons dried onion flakes
1 tablespoon freeze-dried parsley
fresh ground black pepper
2 tablespoons gluten free tamari—or coconut aminos
unfiltered extra virgin olive oil

Instructions

Place a doubled-up piece of aluminum foil into a baking pan. The piece needs to be long enough to completely enclose 3 large (1 lb each) bone-in chicken breasts, or 6-7 small breasts (about 3lbs of raw chicken weight with skin and bones) in a tightly sealed foil packet. Place breasts rib side up. Smear each breast with 1/3 of the bouillon paste. Just smear the rib side and don't worry about doing the meat/skin side. (That's face down on the foil sheet, remember?)

Sprinkle both sides of the breast liberally with granulated garlic, minced onion and fresh ground black pepper. Sprinkle breasts with gluten free tamari, fermented soy sauce, or coconut aminos and extra virgin olive oil. Wrap foil tightly to seal chicken and spices in a foil cocoon and place in a roasting pan.

Place roasting pan in the center of the oven and cook at 300° for 1 1/2 to 2 hours. When you think it's done, carefully unseal one end of the foil and take a temperature reading. It should be at least 170°-175° in the thickest part. If done, remove chicken from oven and open foil package. There will be a LOT of super flavorful pan juices. Save the pan juices to dip the chicken in or to make gravy, soup, stew or barbecue sauce.

Cool chicken until it's cool enough to work with (about 15-20 minutes). Pull, tear or cut chicken into chunks or slices. Place in a container. Cover with about 1/3-1/2 cup of the pan juices. When completely cool, store in an airtight container up to 5 days—or portion and freeze in 4-6 ounce portions. Remember to B/T (bag 'n' tag)! Enjoy.

Notes

With bone-in chicken breast for as low as $0.89 to $0.99/lb, this meal is a bargain and produces a bonanza of moist, flavor-packed, low carb chicken breasts to use for many different dishes, or as a stand-alone simple protein.

Serving Ideas; Use this chicken throughout the week to replace where you might use rotisserie or baked chicken. It makes great Lucky Leftovers when used as the meat base in many types of dishes from soups, salads, sandwiches and wraps, to casseroles and main attractions!

Nutritional Information

Per Ounce (cooked meat only): 69 Calories; 3g Fat (44.5% calories from fat); 9g Protein; 0.53g Carbohydrate; 0.03g trace Dietary Fiber; 24mg Cholesterol; 0.5g Effective Carbs

3 Ounces (cooked meat only): 206 Calories; 10g Fat (44.5% calories from fat); 26g Protein; 1.58g Carbohydrate; 0.08g trace Dietary Fiber; 73mg Cholesterol; 1.5g Effective Carbs

4 Ounces (cooked meat only): 275 Calories; 13g Fat (44.5% calories from fat); 35g Protein; 2.11g Carbohydrate; 0.11g Dietary Fiber; 2g Effective Carbs; 2g Effective Carbs

CHAPTER 3- KETO RECIPES FOR DINNER

Looking to keep it low-carb for dinner? Look no further! Whether you're doing the keto diet for weight loss or healing – or you're just feeling like you need a little cleanse from the starch – these low-carb, keto dinners are worthy of going into the nightly rotation.

Caprese hasselback chicken

I recently found a new hobby when I make chicken recipes. I normally stuff or roll chicken breasts and thighs with different ingredients, but since Hasselback everything has been quite popular these days, I decided to make some Hasselback Chicken Caprese. If you're not familiar with Hasselback cooking, it's essentially a different way to stuff a chicken breast by making slits into the chicken breasts (or meat, potatoes, carrots, zucchinis). I added a bit of homemade pesto and black olives because those are two of my favourite things in the world!!

I think this dish is the easiest thing to make when you're pressed on time or if you don't feel like being in the kitchen too long. In this recipe, I actually used some goat fresh mozzarella cheese, but you can use any type of mozzarella. I prefer using skinless chicken breasts just because it's easier to slit, but you could use breasts with skin and slit the breasts on the opposite side and bake the breasts skin side down. I used some fresh basil from my garden, a few black olives and a tomato.

I personally prefer to use a cast iron skillet to make these because it cooks the meat evenly, but you could use any type of oven bakeware you have. To make Hasselback chicken, all you need to do is slit the chicken breasts. I personally put about 1cm between each cut, but you can definitely make the cuts thicker. I then rubbed a tablespoon of pesto sauce in between each slices and filled each slices randomly with the cheese, tomatoes, olives and basil leaves. I add a bit of olive oil to a cast iron skillet, place the breasts in and sprinkle some salt and pepper over. Just bake and they are done! The breasts end up extremely juicy because they cook in their own juice.

Prep Time 10 minutes
Cook Time 22 minutes
Total Time 32 minutes
Servings 2 people

Calories 552 kcal

Ingredients

2 skinless chicken breasts 500g

2 tbsp homemade pesto or switch to a basil base one

1 tomato

10 black olives

100 g fresh goat mozzarella cheese

30 leaves fresh basil

1/4 tsp Himalayan salt

1/4 tsp black pepper

1 tbsp extra virgin olive oil

Instructions

Preheat the oven to 200C/400F.

Slice the tomato and cut each slice in half. Slice the black olives in half.

Slice the mozzarella into 10 slices. Take the stems off the basil.

Using a sharp knife, make slits in the chicken breasts that are about 1cm wide, making sure not to cut all the way down through the bottom of the chicken breast.

Brush a tbsp of pesto inside each slit of each breast. Stuff the breasts, randomly, with the cheese, tomatoes, olives and basil.

Add the olive oil to the bottom of a cast iron skillet and carefully place the chicken breasts over. Sprinkle the salt and pepper over each breast. Place in the oven and bake for 22 minutes.

Nutrition Facts

Amount Per Serving (1 person)
Calories 552 Calories from Fat 245
% Daily Value*
Total Fat 27.21g 42%
Saturated Fat 8.26g 41%
Cholesterol 181mg 60%
Sodium 471mg 20%
Total Carbohydrates 5.29g 2%
Dietary Fiber 1.7g 7%
Sugars 1.76g
Protein 67.78g 136%
* Percent Daily Values are based on a 2000 calorie diet.

Cabbage lasagna

prep time:40 minutes

cook time:20 minutes

total time:60 minutes

makes 8 -10 servings

If carbs made us skinny, we'd wither away to nothing. This fabulous low-carb cabbage lasagna recipe is a protein-packed adventure minus all the guilt.

Ingredients

2 medium-sized cabbages

2 lbs lean ground beef

28 oz can tomatoes, crushed

1 Anaheim pepper, chopped

1 clove garlic, minced

1 yellow onion, or white, finely chopped

1 tsp oregano

2 tsp basil

1 egg whites

1 cup Gouda cheese, shredded

1 cup mozzarella cheese, shredded

1 cup Parmesan cheese, shredded

salt and pepper, to taste

red pepper flakes

Instruction

Preheat oven to 375 degrees.

Cut cabbage heads in half and boil for 15-20 minutes until soft. Drain water and chop into 1" squares. Then sauté cabbage for 2-3 minutes to remove excess water. Let cool and wrap cabbage leaves in dishtowel squeezing out remaining water.

Brown beef in skillet. When most of the pink is gone, add pepper and onion. Saute 3 more minutes until thoroughly cooked and onion has softened. Add garlic, oregano and basil and cook 1 more minute. Remove from heat.

In a medium bowl whisk egg white into crushed tomatoes. Add to meat mixture and season with salt and pepper.

In a separate bowl mix cheeses together.

To assemble, double layer cabbage, meat sauce, and cheese in greased 9" x 13" pan. Sprinkle with red pepper flakes if desired. Bake 20 minutes or until golden brown

Low-Carb Zucchini Nachos

Recipe type: Type: Paleo, Gluten-free, Dairy-free, Sugar-free, Grain-free, Nut-free, Egg-free, Low-carb, Keto

Prep time: 20 mins Cook time: 30 mins Total time: 50 mins

Serves: 2

Disks of crisp zucchini slices topped with spicy beef, olives, green onions and dairy-free cheese. Served alongside MCT guacamole enriched with Vital Proteins Collagen Peptides. MACROS Fat 60% Carbs 10% Protein 30%.

Ingredients
Low-Carb Nacho Chips
2 medium zucchini, sliced into thin rounds
Meat
½ pound (225 g) regular ground beef
½ tablespoon chili powder

½ teaspoon finely ground gray sea salt

½ teaspoon paprika

½ teaspoon ground cumin

¼ teaspoon garlic powder

¼ teaspoon onion powder

¼ teaspoon crushed red pepper flakes

¼ teaspoon dried oregano leaves

MCT Guacamole

1 avocado

2 tablespoons Vital Proteins Collagen Peptides

1 tablespoon MCT oil

1 tablespoon apple cider vinegar

½ teaspoon dried oregano

¼ teaspoon finely ground gray sea salt

pinch vitamin C crystals, optional

Toppings

⅓ cup (38 g) shredded dairy-free cheese, optional

3 tablespoons sliced black olives

2 green onions, sliced

Instructions

Line a large plate with parchment paper, placing each of the zucchini disks onto the paper being sure to not overlap. You will have to cook the zucchini in batches.

Transfer the plate to the microwave and cook for 8 to 10 minutes on 50% power setting. You know the chips will be done with the edges curl and the middles get slightly golden. Once complete, remove the parchment paper from the microwave, flip over, and drop the chips onto a cooling rack. Repeat with remaining zucchini rounds.

Meanwhile, place all the meat ingredients into a large frying pan. Heat on medium, rotating until the meat is no longer pink.

Combine all of the MCT Guacamole ingredients together in a medium-sized bowl. Mash until combined.

Transfer to a clean plate. Top with cooked meat, cheese, olives, and sliced green onions. Serve alongside MCT guacamole.

Notes

Paleo: to keep the recipe paleo, remove the dairy-free cheese.

Nutrition Information Per Serving

Calories: 578
Total Fat: 38.6

Saturated Fat: 9.1 g

Cholesterol: 101> mg

Sodium: 835 mg

Carbs: 16.4 g

Dietary Fiber: 9.1 g

Net Carbs: 7.3 g

Sugars: 1.3 g

Protein: 43.7 g

Steak kebabs chimichurri sauce

My favorite way to eat steak is topped with this AWESOME chimichurri sauce! It adds flavor and zing to anything you're grilling!

INGREDIENTS:

1 1/4 pounds beef, (sirloin or Angus) cut into 1-inch cubes

fresh ground pepper

1 1/4 tsp kosher salt

1 large red onion, cut into large chunks

18 cherry tomatoes

6 bamboo skewers, soaked in water for 1 hour

FOR THE CHIMICHURRI SAUCE:

2 packed tbsp parsley, finely chopped (no stems)
2 packed tbsp chopped cilantro
2 tbsp red onion, finely chopped
1 clove garlic, minced
2 tbsp extra virgin olive oil
2 tbsp apple cider vinegar
1 tbsp water
1/4 tsp kosher salt
1/8 tsp fresh black pepper
1/8 tsp crushed red pepper flakes, or more to taste

DIRECTIONS:

Season the meat with salt and pepper.

For the chimichurri, combine the red onion, vinegar, salt and olive oil and let it sit for about 5 minutes. Add the remaining ingredients and mix; set aside in the refrigerator until ready to use (can be made a few hours ahead).

Place the onions, beef and tomatoes onto the skewers.

Prepare the grill on high heat. Grill the steaks to desired doneness, about 2 to 3 minutes per side for medium-rare. Transfer steaks to a platter and top with chimichurri sauce.

NUTRITION INFORMATION

Calories: 219

Total Fat: 13g

Saturated Fat: g

Cholesterol: 62.5mg

Sodium: 335.5mg

Carbohydrates: 5.5g

Fiber: 1g

Sugar: 0g

Protein: 20g

Keto Reuben Stromboli

Delicious buttery keto pastry dough wrapped around the fillings of a classic Reuben sandwich. And sugar-free Russian dressing to dip it in too! This is the stuff my low carb dreams are made of.

INGREDIENTS

1 recipe Magic Mozzarella dough
1 20ounces corned beef, chopped
4 ounces thinly sliced Swiss cheese
1 cup sauerkraut, well drained
2 tsp caraway seeds

SUGAR-FREE RUSSIAN DRESSING

1/3 cup mayonnaise
2 tbsp finely diced dill pickle
1 tbsp tomato paste
2 tsp Swerve Sweetener
1/4 tsp ground cumin
1/8 tsp ground cloves

INSTRUCTIONS

Preheat the oven to 350F. Follow the directions to make the dough. Brush a large piece of parchment paper or a silicone liner with oil and turn out the dough onto this surface.

Cover with another piece of parchment and roll out to a 16x10 inch rectangle. Cut strips on the diagonal down the long sides of the rectangle, about 1 inch wide and 3 inches long.

Mound the chopped corned beef down the center of the rectangle. Top with slices of Swiss cheese and the sauerkraut.

Fold the strips of dough over the filling so that the ends overlap. Pinch the dough on the ends to seal. Sprinkle the top with caraway seeds and press lightly to adhere.

Bake 25 to 35 minutes, until the dough is golden brown. Remove and let cool at least 15 minutes before slicing.

SUGAR-FREE RUSSIAN DRESSING:

In a medium bowl, whisk together the mayo, pickle, tomato paste, sweetener, cumin, and cloves. Serve on the side with the stromboli.

by Carolyn

RECIPE NOTES

Serves 8 (stromboli + dressing). Each serving has 4.16g NET CARBS.

Stromboli per serving: Food energy: 349kcal Total fat: 25.63g Calories from fat: 230 Cholesterol: 90mg Carbohydrate: 6.31g Total dietary fiber: 2.63g Protein: 18.97g

Russian Dressing per serving: Food energy: 71kcal Total fat: 7.44g Calories from fat: 66 Cholesterol: -- Carbohydrate: 0.67g Total dietary fiber: 0.19g Protein: 0.14g

Spinach Tomato Meatza Pizza - Paleo Low Carb

A paleo friendly low carb pizza with seasoned ground beef mix cooked flat to make a crust. Then, it's topped off with veggies.

Prep Time 8 minutes
Cook Time 22 minutes
Total Time 30 minutes
Servings 8 servings
Calories 344 kcal

Ingredients
2 eggs
1/2 cup parmesan cheese grated
2 teaspoons Italian seasonings
1 teaspoon garlic powder
1 teaspoon salt
2 pounds ground beef
2 tomatoes

9 ounces frozen chopped spinach cooked and drained
2 cups mozzarella cheese shredded

Instructions

Beat the eggs with the parmesan cheese and all seasonings.
Add the ground beef and mix until well combined.
Spread the mixture onto a large baking sheet with sides (a jelly roll pan works well).

The mix doesn't have to fill the bottom of the pan, I made rounded ends.

Bake for about 20 minutes in a 450 degree F oven.
Remove from oven and drain off any grease.
Place sliced tomatoes and spinach on top then sprinkle with mozzarella cheese.

Return to oven on a high rack near broiler. Broil until cheese is melted and brown.

Recipe Notes
Use cheese alternative for paleo.

Net carbs per serving: 3g

Nutrition Facts

Spinach Tomato Meatza Pizza - Paleo Low Carb

Amount Per Serving (296 g)

Calories 344 Calories from Fat 134

% Daily Value*

Total Fat 14.9g 23%

Saturated Fat 7.1g 36%

Cholesterol 162mg 54%

Sodium 643mg 27%

Potassium 730mg 21%

Total Carbohydrates 4.1g 1%

Dietary Fiber 1.2g 5%

Sugars 1.1g

Protein 47.3g 95%

Vitamin A 67%

Vitamin C 22%

Calcium 13%

Iron 125%

* Percent Daily Values are based on a 2000 calorie diet.

Bacon cheeseburger casserole

YIELD: SERVES 6

PREP TIME: 30 MINUTES COOK TIME: 30 MINUTES

TOTAL TIME: 1 HOUR

INGREDIENTS:

1/2 pound bacon

1 pound ground beef

1/2 sweet onion

1 clove garlic

4 tablespoons cream cheese

2 tablespoons reduced sugar ketchup

1 tablespoon yellow mustard

1 tablespoon Worcestershire sauce

1 teaspoon seasoned salt

4 large eggs

1/4 cup heavy cream

1 teaspoon ground pepper

1 teaspoon hot sauce

8 ounces grated cheddar

1 teaspoon fresh dill

DIRECTIONS:

Dice the bacon into small pieces and place in a large skillet over medium heat. Cook, stirring often, until crisp. Remove bacon from pan and set aside. Drain grease from pan.

Add the ground beef to the skillet and cook until browned, crumbling as it cooks. Drain fat.

Add the onion and garlic to the skillet with the beef and cook until translucent, about 5 minutes.

Add the cream cheese, ketchup, mustard, Worcestershire sauce, and seasoned salt to the skillet and cook over low heat, stirring constantly, until combined.

Spread the beef mixture into a greased 8x8 baking dish. Top with the cooked bacon.

Crack the eggs into a medium bowl and whisk together with the heavy cream until combined. Stir in the pepper and hot sauce.

Pour the egg mixture over the beef and bacon.

Top with the cheddar cheese.

Bake at 350 degrees for 30 minutes or until set and golden on top. Sprinkle with dill before serving.

Nutrition Facts

Serving Size

Servings Per Container 6

Amount Per Serving

Calories 582 Calories from Fat 387

% Daily Value*

Total Fat 43g 66%

Saturated Fat 22g 110%

Trans Fat 0g

Cholesterol 237mg 79%

Sodium 1891mg 79%

Total Carbohydrate 2g 1%

Dietary Fiber 0g 0%

Sugars 1g

Protein 43g 86%

ABOUT THE AUTHOR

David D. Kings is an experienced chef and nutritionist; Kings has years of experience helping people learn to eat better, lose weight, become fit and live a healthier life.

David D. Kings

ONE LAST THING...

If you enjoyed this book or found it useful, I'd be very grateful if you'd post a short review on Amazon. Your support really does make a difference, and I read all the reviews personally so I can get your feedback and make this book even better.

Thanks again for your support!

Made in the USA
San Bernardino, CA
23 November 2017